To:

From:

Art Direction: Trinidad Vergara
Design: Renata Biernat
Photography of the artwork: © Superstock
Literary Research:
María Eugenia Díaz Cafferata
Enriqueta Naón Roca

www.vergarariba.com

ISBN: 987-9338-64-2

Printed in Singapore

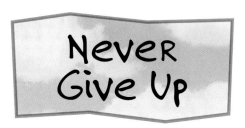

Never Give Up

Edited by Lidia María Riba

V&R
PUBLISHERS

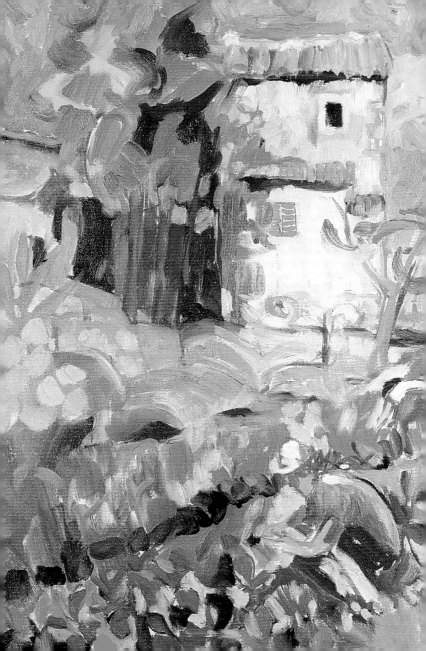

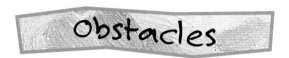

Obstacles

Look to this day, for it is life,
The very life of life. In its brief
Course lie all the realities and
Verities of existence; the bliss of growth,
The splendor of action, the glory of power . . .

For yesterday is but a dream,
And tomorrow is only
A vision, but today, well lived,
Makes every yesterday a dream of happiness
And every tomorrow a vision of hope.

Old Sanskrit Text

Jump into the middle of things, get your hands dirty, fall flat on your face, and then, reach for the stars.

Joan L. Curcio

Sweat: to sprinkle history. Pain: to cultivate life.

Antonio Gracia

Opposition is not a stone in the middle of your path.
It is up to you to transform it into a stepping-stone
that will take you higher.

Franco Molinari

The greater the obstacle, the greater the glory
of overcoming it.

Molière

I will never defend pain and it is the obligation of everyone who considers himself human to collaborate in its elimination. But I will say that those who suffer come to possess the potential of knowing how to create and that, from pain, strength is gained to develop life.

J. Borão

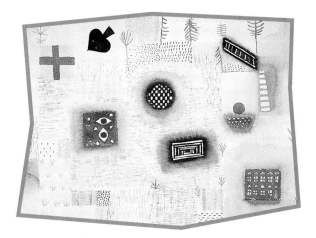

Some defeats have more dignity than victory itself.

Jorge Luis Borges

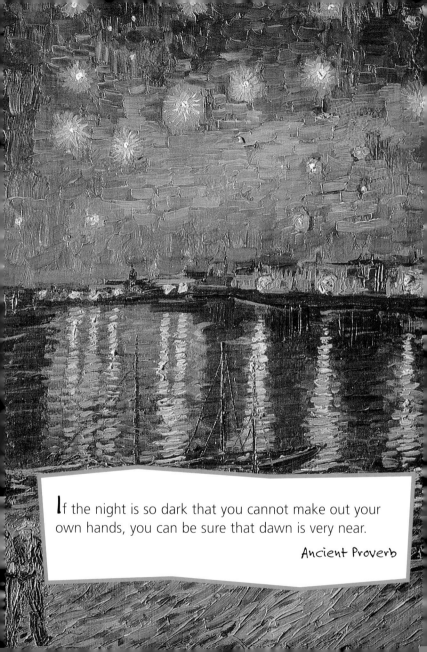

If the night is so dark that you cannot make out your own hands, you can be sure that dawn is very near.

Ancient Proverb

The road to success is always under construction.

Lily Tomlin

Nothing stops the man who desires to achieve. Every obstacle is simply a cause to develop his achievement muscle.

Eric Butterworth

The present is nothing but the attempt of the past to become the future.

Miguel de Unamuno

You may be disappointed if you fail, but you are doomed if you don't try.

Beverly Sills

How happy we would be if we took away the tensions, if we assumed the best, if the future were our goal. Perhaps then we would better understand that in our hearts is a field where the seeds of tomorrow have been sown. And there would be reason to thank those who venture forth with doubts and in risk, those who blaze the path toward the unknown.

Antonio Alonso

How often we withdraw into ourselves to take refuge! And yet our weapons are within: the golden wings of intelligence, the iron shield of willpower, the jousting spear of words, the red sandals of courage. How infrequently we bare our souls!

José Luis Martín Descalzo

We fear success as much as we fear failure.
The difference is that the fear of failure is obvious, while the fear of success is hidden and can therefore do more damage. It behooves us to bring it out of the darkness to tackle it straight on.

Carlos González Valles

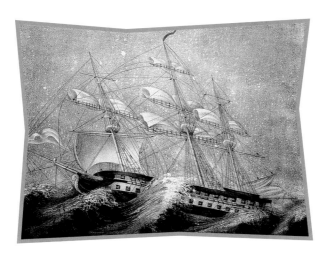

Fishermen know that the sea is dangerous and storms terrible. But that knowledge does not stop them from setting sail.

Vincent Van Gogh

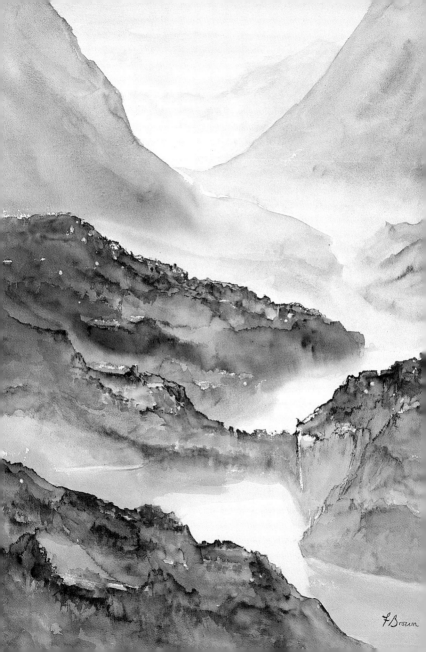

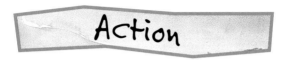

Action

You are the profound desire that propels you.
As your desire is, so is your will.
As your will is, so are your acts.
As are your acts, so will your destiny be.

Brihadaranyaka Upanishad

Our greatest weakness lies in giving up. The most
certain way to succeed is to always try one more time.

Thomas A. Edison

To be a realist, you must believe in miracles.

David Ben Gurion

Make up your mind to act decidedly and take the consequences.
No good is ever done in this world by hesitation.

Thomas Henry Huxley

All our dreams can come true, if we have the desire to pursue them.

Walt Disney

What one has, one ought to use; and whatever he does, he should do with all his might.

Cicero

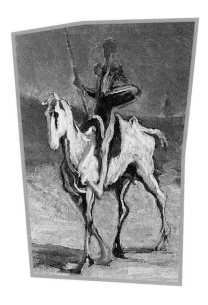

The only way to discover the limits of the possible is to go beyond them into the impossible.

Arthur C. Clarke

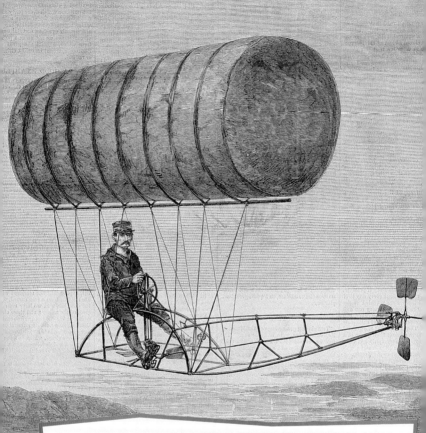

Even if strength fails, boldness at least will deserve praise: in great endeavours even to have had the will is enough.

Protagoras

Imagination has always had powers of resurrection that no science can match.

Ingrid Bengis

I sought advice and cooperation from all those around me, but never permission.

Muhammad Ali

My mother suggested I wrote a story to relieve the boredom when I was sick and I told her I didn't know how. "How do you know if you have never tried?" she asked.

Agatha Christie

Tell me not in mournful numbers,
Life is but an empty dream!
For the soul is dead that slumbers,
And things are not what they seem.

Lives of great men all remind us
We can make our lives sublime.
And departing, leave behind us
Footprints on the sands of time.

Let us then, be up and doing
With a heart for any fate;
Still achieving, still pursuing,
Learn to labor and to wait.

Henry W. Longfellow

A life spent making mistakes is not only
more honorable but more useful than a life
spent doing nothing.

George Bernard Shaw

The true journey of discovery is not looking for new lands, but looking with new eyes.

Marcel Proust

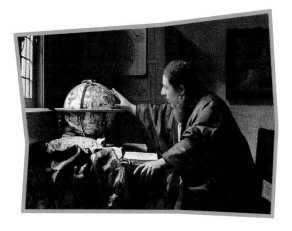

There are other worlds, but they are in this one.

Paul Eluard

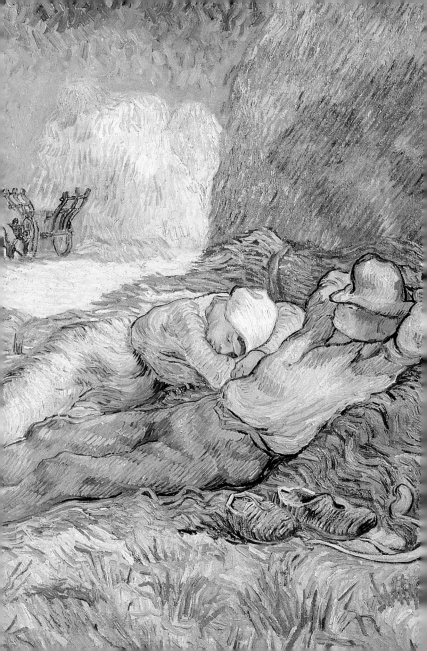

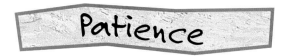

Patience

It takes twenty years to make an overnight success.

Eddie Cantor

There is always something to make you wonder, in the shape of a leaf, the trembling of a tree.

Albert Schweitzer

Do what you can, with what you have, where you are.

Theodore Roosevelt

Utopia is on the horizon. I come two steps closer, it moves two steps away. I walk ten steps and the horizon runs ten steps farther. That is what utopia is for: walking.

Eduardo Galeano

On no account brood over your wrongdoing. Rolling in the muck is not the best way of getting clean.

Aldous Huxley

If you wish success in life, make perseverance your bosom friend, experience your wise counselor, caution your elder brother and hope your guardian genius.

Joseph Addison

Wisely and slow; they stumble that run fast.

William Shakespeare

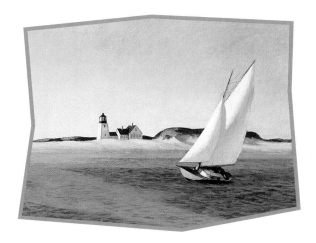

Progress is comparatively slow. We must be satisfied to advance in life as we walk, step by step.

Samuel Smiles

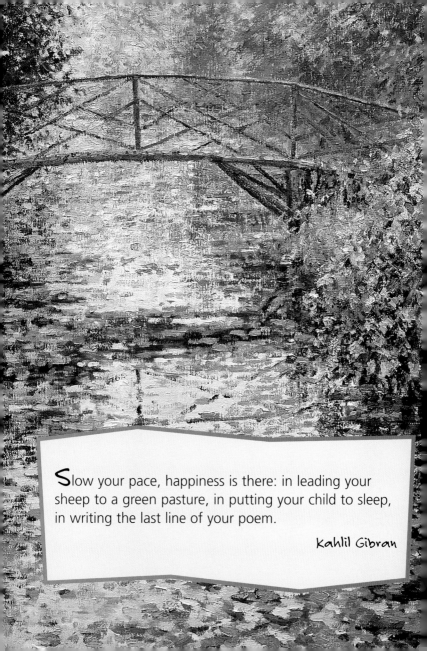

Slow your pace, happiness is there: in leading your sheep to a green pasture, in putting your child to sleep, in writing the last line of your poem.

Kahlil Gibran

Give me a soul that is never bored,
that has no complaints, frustrations nor quarrels.
Father, grant me a sense of humor,
give me the grace to take a joke,
to have a little bit of happiness in life
and to share it with others.

Sir Thomas More

Allow me to tell you the secret that helped me
reach my goals.
My strength resides solely in my tenacity.

Louis Pasteur

You just can't beat the person who never gives up!

Babe Ruth

Never enumerate what you are missing. Do count all that you have. You will see, in sum, that life has been magnificent to you.

Amado Nervo

God hears us when nothing responds. He is within us when we think we are alone. He calls us when we are abandoned.

St. Augustine

It does not matter how slowly you go, so long as you do not stop.

Confucius

There is no need to leave the room. It is enough to sit down at the table and listen. It is not even necessary to listen, just wait. You don't even have to wait, just learn to be silent. The world will offer itself to you liberally to be discovered.

Franz Kafka

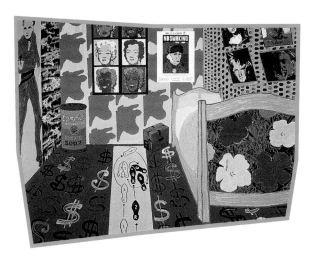

A free man is by necessity insecure; a thinking man by necessity, uncertain.

Erich Fromm

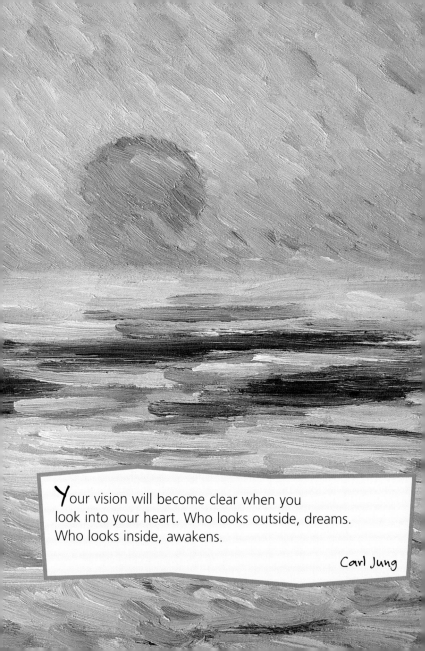

Your vision will become clear when you look into your heart. Who looks outside, dreams. Who looks inside, awakens.

Carl Jung

When you are inspired by some great purpose, some extraordinary project, all your thoughts break their bounds. Dormant forces, faculties and talents become alive, and you discover yourself a greater person. Your mind trascends limitations.

Patanjali

There is nothing softer or more yielding than water, yet nothing is better at conquering the unyielding rock. Weakness overcomes strength and gentleness overcomes rigidity.

Lao Tzu

If I have made any valuable discoveries,
it has been owing more to patient attention,
than to any other talent.

Sir Isaac Newton

To finish first you must first finish.

Rick Mears

Diamonds are only chunks of coal that stuck
to their jobs.

Minnie Richards Smith

There are simple things that have far-reaching effects. One of them is contemplating the stars from the solitude of a mountain.

Francisco García

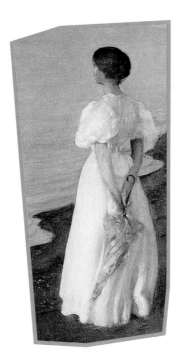

Go for what has inspired you and be patient.

The Koran

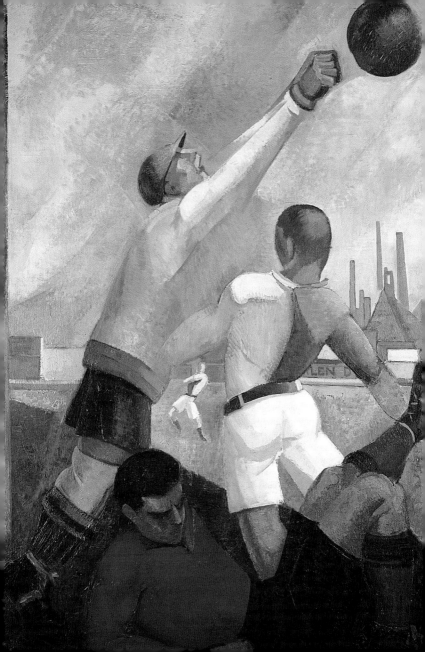

Triumph

History has demonstrated that the most notable winners usually encountered heartbreaking obstacles before they triumphed. They won because they refused to become discouraged by their defeats.

B. C. Forbes

Nothing is as real as a dream. And if you go for it, something really good is going to happen to you. You may grow old but you never really get old.

Tom Clancy

Some men give up when they have almost reached their goal; while others, on the contrary, obtain victory by exerting at the last moment, more vigorous efforts than before.

Polybius

What you do is more important than how much you make, and how you feel about it is more important than what you do.

Jerry Gilles

What is important is to keep learning, to enjoy challenge, and to tolerate ambiguity. In the end there are no certain answers.

Marina Horner

There must be a beginning of any great matter, but the continuing unto the end until it be thoroughly finished yields the true glory.

Sir Francis Drake

Up to a point, a man's life is shaped by environment, heredity, and changes in the world about him; then comes a time when it lies within his grasp to shape the clay of his life into the sort of thing he wishes to be... Everyone has it within his power to say, *this I am today, that I shall be tomorrow*.

Louis L'Amour

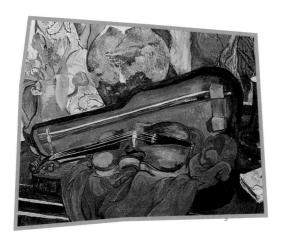

Why be a man when you can be a success?

Bertolt Brecht

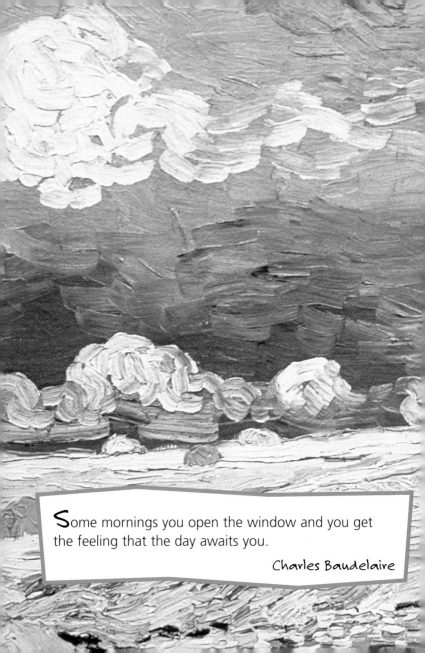

Some mornings you open the window and you get the feeling that the day awaits you.

Charles Baudelaire

The joyfulness of a man prolongeth his days.

Psalms

Come my friends,
Tis not too late
To seek a newer world.

Alfred, Lord Tennyson

If I have been able to see farther than others, it is
because I have stood on the shoulders of giants.

Sir Isaac Newton

I will always prefer dreamers… even if they're wrong; those who hope… even if their hopes sometimes fall through; those who are pursuing utopia… even if they end up stranded mid-stream. I bet on those who trust that the world can and should change; those who believe in future happiness. The kingdom of happiness will be only for those with hope.

José Luis Martín Descalzo

He who is fixed to a star does not change his mind.

Leonardo Da Vinci

The gloom of the world is but a shadow. Behind it, yet within our reach, is joy. There is radiance and glory in the darkness, could we see; and to see, we have only to look.

Fra Giovanni

A man likes marvelous things; so he invents them, and is astonished.

Edgar Watson Howe

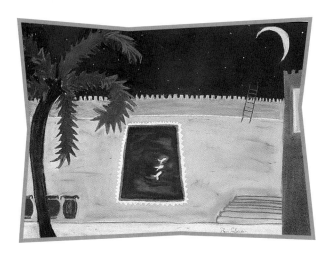

My formula for success?
Rise early, work late, strike oil.

Jean Paul Getty

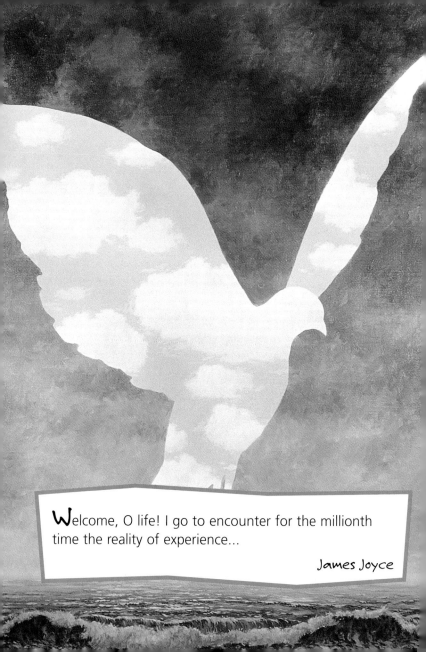

Welcome, O life! I go to encounter for the millionth time the reality of experience...

James Joyce

No coward soul is mine,
No trembler in the world's storm-troubled sphere:
I see Heaven's glories shine,
And faith shines equal,
Arming me from fear.

Emily Brontë

We were born to fly and we have an obligation
to attempt to soar again and again. I can tell you
that I have crashed and broken apart many times.
But I persist. When you feel you are collapsing,
that you're falling into faintness between
splinters and bones, between flames of sand and
showers of glass, beat your wings. And up again.

Jesús Quintero

Paintings Reproduced in this Book:

Cover and page 42: *The Great Family* - René Magritte (1898-1967),
     Private Collection.
Page 6:   *Bean Harvesters* - Josephine Trotter (1940-).
Page 9:   *Garden Signs* - Paul Klee (1879-1940), Barnes Foundation,
     Merion, Pennsylvania.
Page 10: *Starry Night over the River* - Vincent Van Gogh (1853-1890),
     Musée d'Orsay, Paris.
Page 13: *Storm at Cape Horn* - Nath & James Currier & Ives
     (1857-1907), Library of Congress, Washington, D.C.
Page 14: *Misty River* - Florence Brown Eden, Contemporary Gallery,
     Jacksonville, Florida.
Page 17: *Don Quixote* - Honoré Daumier (1808-1879).
Page 18: *Gas Propelled Aircraft* - Unknown Artist.
Page 21: *The Astronomer* - Jan Vermeer (1632-1675), Musée du Louvre,
     Paris.
Page 22: *Noon, Rest from Work* - Vincent Van Gogh (1853-1890),
     Musée d'Orsay, Paris.
Page 25: *Long Leg* - Edward Hopper (1882-1967), The Huntington
     Library, Art Collections & Botanical Gardens, San Marino, CA.
Page 26: *Water Lilies and Japanese Bridge* - Charles Neal (1951-),
     Byfleet Manor, Surrey.
Page 29: *Andy's Gone* - Tsing-Fang Chen (1930-), Lucia Gallery,
     New York.
Page 30: *Sun Reflections on the Sea* - Nicholas Tarkoff (1871-1930),
     Images of Christie's, New York.
Page 33: *Evening Splendor* - Charles Courtney Curran (1861-1942),
     Images of Christie's, New York.
Page 34: *Players on the Field* - Angel Zarraga (1886-1946),
     Images of Christie's, New York.
Page 37: *The Violin Case* - Suzanne Valadon (1867-1938),
     Musée de l'Art Modern de la Ville de Paris.
Page 38: *Field under Storm Clouds* - Vincent Van Gogh (1853-1890),
     Van Gogh Museum, Amsterdam.
Page 41: *Swimming to the Moon:* # 2 of a series - Sherri Silverman,
     Private Collection.